![barcode] I0022734

SomaVeda™
Integrated Traditional Therapies

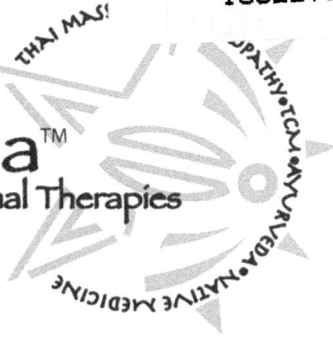

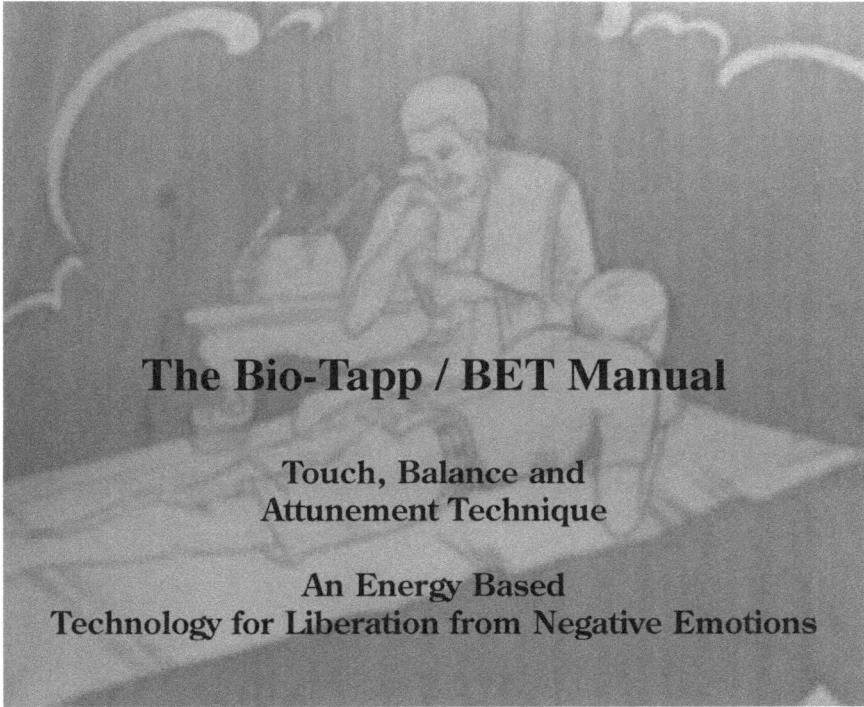

The Bio-Tapp / BET Manual

Touch, Balance and
Attunement Technique

An Energy Based
Technology for Liberation from Negative Emotions

By

Anthony B. James
DNM, ND(T), MD(AM), DOM, RAAP

Aachan and Master teacher of SomaVeda Thai Yoga

The Bio-Tapp / BET Manual

Touch, Balance and Attunement Technique

An Energy Based Technology
for Liberation from Negative Emotions

By

Anthony B. James DNM, ND(T), MD(AM), DOM, RAAP

Aachan and Master teacher of SomaVeda® Thai Yoga

The Use of Bio Neuro Harmonics: Adaptive Resonant Field Adjustment Incorporating Emotional Liberation Technique (Bio-Tapp/ B.E.T.) to support the Human Biological Transformational Apparatus. Otherwise known as "The Machine".

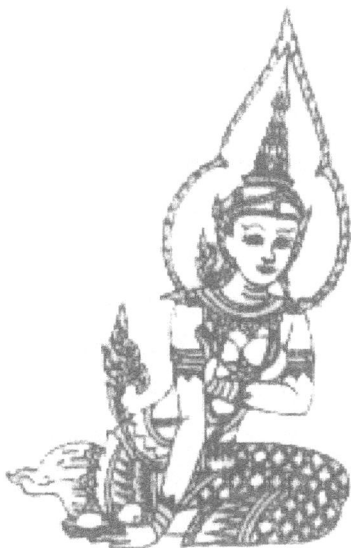

The Bio-Tapp/BET Manual

Anthony B. James, DNM, ND(T), MD(AM), DOM, RAAP

Copyright © 2010 by Anthony B. James

Inquires should be addressed to:

Anthony B. James, DNM, ND(T), MD(AM), DOM, RAAP
5401 Saving Grace Ln. Brooksville, FL 34602
(706) 358- 8646
Email: itta@core.com
Website: http://www.ThaiYogaCenter.Com

Meta Journal Press
ISBN: 978-1-886338-24-1 (Trade Paper)
Original Manuscript Copyright Date: February 2010
Published Perfect Bound Edition 2010

Printed in the U.S.A
Cover Illustration by Anthony B. James
Original art and photography by Anthony B. James
Typography by Anthony B. James
Design art and original design by Anthony B. James

EVAL

52088

9 781886 338241

Dedication

This book is dedicated to my wife and fellow vision holder Julie James and to all of my teachers and students who have over the years opened my eyes to all of the endless possibilities of what SomaVeda Integrated Traditional Therapies based on Thai Yoga and Thai Massage have to offer for reducing suffering and supporting joyful life in the world.

As quoted from the Buddha "man must himself rise and open the portals that give upon liberty, and neither are those portals locked and the keys in posession of someone from whom they must be obtained by prayer and entreaty, that door is free of all bolts and bars save thove that man himself has made. (Piyadassi Thera)

Acknowledgement

I want to give a special acknowledgement to several individuals who made substantial contributions to my knowledge and appreciation of the use of tapping for healing. First, we have come a long way from the original Chinese and Tibetan Organ, Meridian, Five Element and Acupoint tapping protocols first taught me in the 80's by Sensei Kiku Miyasaki and Toshiko Phipps and my Thai teachers Phraa Khruu Men, Phrakhru Uppakarn Phatanakit, Aachan Boontum Kitniwan (Nuad Thai), Khruu Vilawong Sidtisopong. However, this is where my appreciation and use of tapping energy points and lines was first discovered and I give credit to them for bringing the idea of tapping acupuncture points, Lom, Marma and Chakra to all of us.

Second, to Gary Craig the founder and innovator of the EFT, Emotional Freedom Technique for his contribution and permission to incorporate elements derived from the EFT protocol into our treatment strategy. In particular his "Basic Recipe" as shown later in this manual has been a great asset in simplifying the practical aspects of doing and applying these principles simply and without the need for a wooden hammer!

Although, this EFT oriented book is provided as a good faith effort to expand the use of EFT and related concepts and practices in the world. "The Bio-Tapp/ BET Manual" represents the unique ideas, innovations, understandings of SomaVeda, Integrated Traditional Therapies and the author, Anthony B. James and does not necessarily represent the complete, standardized EFT training offered at http://www.emofree.com".

The Bio-Tapp/BET Manual

SomaVeda® Bio-Tapp/B.E.T. Can bring relief from all issues such as...

Chronic Pain	Emotional Disorders
Stress Issues	Confusion
Anger Issues	Dyslexia
Addictions Issues	Claustrophobia
Food Issues	Abuse Issues
Weight Loss Issues	Sports Performance Issues
Anxiety Issues	Bipolar Issues
Trauma Issues	Fear of flying Issues
Allergy Issues	Healing Issues
Depression Issues	Asthma
Fears and Phobias	Fibromyalgia
Allergy Issues	Anguish
Respiratory Problems	Violent Tendencies &
Blood Pressure Issues	Rage Issues
Post Traumatic Stress Disorder	Physical Disease
Relationship Issues	Bruxation and TMJ Issues
Women's Issues	Bulimia, Anorexia Issues
Children's Issues	Nervousness
Geriatric Issues	Cravings & Compulsions
School and Performance issues	Toxicity Issues
Fear of Public Speaking Issues	Energy Balance Issues
Sexual Dysfunction	Heart Burn Issues
Serious Diseases (From Hypertension to Cancer)	
Financial Issues	Limited Beliefs
Blocked Energy	

And so much more!

If you can name it, you can BET it!

Table of Contents

What is SomaVeda® Bio-Tapp/BET?
This manual is a starting point.
A Note on Bio-Tapp/BET's surprising physical healings
Please use this work in an ethical fashion with Common Sense!
Common Uses For Bio-Tapp/BET
Dealing with Side Effects
Our Agreement
What are "Bio-transformational Technologies"?
Our Developmental Plateau
The Two Kinds of Human Beings
What kind of man or women is Bio-Tapp/BET for?
A New Definition of Pain
How To Do A SomaVeda® Bio-Tapp/BET Session
Initial Points for Basic SomaVeda® Bio-Tapp/BET Treatment Algorithm
Hand Points for Basic SomaVeda® Bio-Tapp/BET Treatment Algorithm

The Thirty Four Bio-Tapp/BET Premises:
    1: Everything is Energy
    2: Everything is Connected to Everything Else on some level.
    3: We are part of everything.
    4: Everything affects everything else.
    5: We are Stress Adaptive Electrical-Biological Organisms.
    6: Greater fields influence lesser fields.
    7: The shape and function of the tissue is determined by the wave form it models.
    8: Attitudes are like wires, which connect us to events.
    9: Every event or occurrence experienced throughout life is recorded or stored.
    10: It takes energy to store and to preserve information.
    11: It takes energy to make energy!

12: Negative interference patterns are not real!

13: Reduce the many equals increase the one.

14: Accumulated negative wave forms are Karma.

15: Be What You Know.

16: Reducing Harmful External and Internal
Interferences supports the Work.

17: We are working for the past, the now and the future.

18: The work continues after you die.

19: Advanced teaching includes study of symbols.

20: We chose to live and be this experience.

21: The Matrix Body holds the Key to the Invisible
world.

22: We are fundamentally, literally energy.

23: All is God, All is Energy, All is Electrical, All is
Consciousness.

24: Energy precedes physiology.

25: The Cause of All Negative Emotion is Disruption of
the Body's Energy System.

26: We can change physiology by affecting energy.

27: The body is a stress adaptive organism and vehicle
for transformation.

28 We are not the "Machine" nor are we the "Events"
which happen to it!

29: Balance The Fields

30: "I's" equal sources of inference.

31: Everything about you is mechanical, except what is
not!

32: All chronic disorder and disease in the machine is
supported by negative emotion.

33: Where it hurts it ain't!

34: Psychological, Mental illness and Negative
emotions are the same and have the same
causes.

What is SomaVeda® Bio-Tapp/BET?

The acronym BET stands for Bio Neuro Harmonics: Adaptive Resonant Field Adjustment Incorporating Emotional Liberation Tapping Technique to support the Stress Adaptive Human Biological Transformational Apparatus.

Whew! Now you know also why we call it Bio-Tapp/B.E.T.!

It's a methodology for addressing negative emotional issues of any kind, used in conjunction with other energy based healing practices such as SomaVeda Thai Yoga. The technique is very simple in practice. You basically pick an emotional issue to be treated, tap key energy points in specific patterns or algorithms. At the same time right and left brain integration techniques such as humming/ singing and counting are done simultaneously with the tapping.

SomaVeda® Bio-Tapp/B.E.T. may be a miracle for relief and rescue from chronic issues and pain which are resulting from old and unresolved energy issues relating coming from the past. There is now no reason to continue these old patterns and tapes which limit our ability to be present in the here and now.

This manual is a starting point.

This manual is meant to be an introduction to SomaVeda®
Bio-Tapp/B.E.T. It is a companion to our more extensive live
and DVD based SomaVeda® Bio-Tapp/B.E.T. Level One
Certification Course and is NOT intended to be complete
training.

Study this manual and diligently apply BET to yourself and
others and you will likely get immediate, and often profound
results. The beautiful thing about BET as a possibility for
healing and manifesting emotional liberation is that you can
TEST it! As you begin your practice, you will no doubt have
many questions. We encourage you to either keep practicing,
ask your instructor and/or continue your education with level
two, or further. Many questions are either based on experience, communication or level of practice, and are all easily
remedied.

This manual is not intended to answer all questions. It is just
to get you started in a productive direction for your practice.
It is also support for you to begin today to bring healing and
balance, as well as emotional liberation, to those around you.
The best way to learn BET is to practice with real people in
real life. Take counsel and rely on the training and expertise of
those who are ahead of you and keep an open mind.

This method has been developed out the blending of new and
old science. This is a new work and we present it to you for
both evaluation and for the contribution that one day you may
make as well.

So, if you're intrigued by the technology and wish to develop
further, you will need additional training.

A note on Bio-Tapp/BET's surprising physical healings.

BET was originally designed to overhaul and bring an entirely new dimension to the traditional Oriental practice of SomaVeda® Thai Yoga, Massage, traditional Chinese medicine and similar disciplines.

After teaching hundreds of classes and thousands of students over several years, coupled with the personal experience of treating thousands of patients for every imaginable disease and disorder, I realized that what I actually did in session began to take on some "non-traditional" aspects. (I put non-traditional in quotes because in my heart I now believe we are formulating in a profound way, the real secret healing ways that have been stored and hidden in our traditions.)

In the practice of Thai Yoga and of other related "cousins," we teach all about energy, but we do vinyasa, kata or routines. There are treatment forms that follow predetermined patterns for both general and specific health needs. Additionally, we speak of the "Mind/Body connection," but we then poke, prod and manipulate the client in a fairly physical manner. In our traditional treatment systems, there is a great variety of fairly complex assessments, as well as literally thousands of remedies or treatments for all of our illnesses and disease conditions.

It is quite normal for the average person to take between two to four years to basically comprehend one of these complex systems such as Thai Yoga, Acupuncture, Ayurveda or others. Many students and practitioners at advanced levels struggle with their ability to powerfully treat complex disease patterns. We need a simple, elegant solution. We need solutions which follow universal laws and principles and, while also conforming to current views of science.

Perhaps it is my exposure to the modern sciences and desire to reconcile them with my traditional energetic training that I have had this epiphany of a new paradigm. I do have some good role models. There is one in particular, Phaa Khruu Samaii Mesamarn of my Thai training at Buddhai Sawan Institute in Nongkam Thailand. My primary training and original teaching certification in Thai healing arts came from phaa Khruu Samaii. Truth is, even though I still teach most of what he gave to me technique wise, there was something missing.

I had spent much time and energy imagining and designing a simplified system that would honour the traditional work I had been given. I also wanted to honour my gut and intuition that there was a simple and easily accessible way to reverse energy imbalance that could be taught to anyone, be practiced by anyone and which critically met my intellectual criteria for scientific rational. The integration for the Tibetan style tapping which was taught in Thailand, Japan and the US seemed a good solution.

The only problem was that you still needed a fairly sophisticated knowledge of acupuncture points and lines, or the equivalent of Ayurvedic energy such as Lom, Chakra and Prana Nadi. Since there were literally ten thousand points and more lines, the complexity of combinations of using them is literally infinite. Also the use of tools such as the "tapping" hammer still meant you had to have "tools." I realized that most energy balancing treatments actually use very few common points and there is a bit of repetition of point use. For example, you can see books and manuals which show common point combinations for common ailments such as headache or back pain.

I originally decided to use these traditional Thai Yoga and Acupuncture point combinations with the BET concept to develop a short hand energy balancing system. However, after returning from Thailand in December of 2004, I came across the EmoFree.com website and the EFT. Amazing – It was a system and way of working that was extremely concurrent with my understandings of what a new, simplified energy balancing system could be. Now, I'm not one to reinvent the wheel. Gary Craig and company at EmoFree. com had already invested many hours and efforts into their EFT system, and it was elegant. It lacked, however, certain developments and integrations which my original concept SomaVeda® Bio-Tapp/BET possessed, namely, the use in SomaVeda® style Integrated sessions protocols and technical applications. It lacked the energetic theory basis we had developed.

So, I decided to integrate them. The first thing I did was contact Gary Craig. He gave permission for this integration and exchange of ideas, provided that I made it clear that this SomaVeda® Bio-Tapp/BET work represented OUR views and experiences and not necessarily those of Gary Craig, EFT or any other Tapping based system of healing. So there you have it. There is a clear connection between the EFT information and training set of competencies and those of the SomaVeda® Bio-Tapp/BET. I hope that explaining the crossover and integration of these two systems is not confusing. It is meant in the spirit of "Giving Credit Where Credit Is Due."

The system of BET is the practical formulation of the "Secrets" to healing virtually every disease and disorder know to man, especially focusing on the energetic and emotional components. To say it another way, if there is an energetic component or an emotional component to any illness, this method will balance, restore or resolve it. Phaa Khruu and other teachers have told me that it takes less time than to snap the fingers to balance the energy; sometimes, however, it takes longer for us to see the results. When you use this BET, most times the issue will resolve immediately, even instantly, but sometimes it will not. Sometimes it will take a bit longer

based on various factors which we will teach you.
This way of working represents the next evolution in
Oriental and western methods of medicine and healing which
are energetic and/or relate to the emotional well being of
people. The goal of a simple, easily learned and practiced
method will enable virtually anyone to learn how to heal
themselves, their friends, family, clients and patients.

We have found that SomaVeda® Bio-Tapp/BET and similar
systems address causes that Western Healing Practices have
largely ignored. Western Medicine, for example, pays very
little attention to disruptions in the body's energy meridians,
nor does it give much weight to emotional causes. These
causes, of course, are the centerpiece of BET. Thus, it is no
wonder that BET produces benefits where the medical
profession has thrown up its hands. The reason is simply
because we are taking aim at causes that others have largely
disregarded.

Note to physicians, naturopaths, chiropractors, homeopaths,
herbalists, thai yoga practitioners and therapists, massage
therapists, physicians, ministers and other members of the
healing professions: This material may represent a radical de-
parture from conventional techniques that your familiar with.
Properly used, it should multiply your ability to assist both
yourself and others in resolving previously hidden disruptive
energetic and emotional patterns. BET may address
fundamental causes of chronic negative emotional issues.

The Bio-Tapp/ BET protocols are specifically designed to be
used in concert or conjunction with SomaVeda Thai Yoga,
Integrated Traditional Therapies. Even though they are
specifically designed for this purpose they can be used as
stand alone techniques for healing anytime, anywhere.
Additionally they can be integrated into effective use into
almost any other type of medical and or healing work.

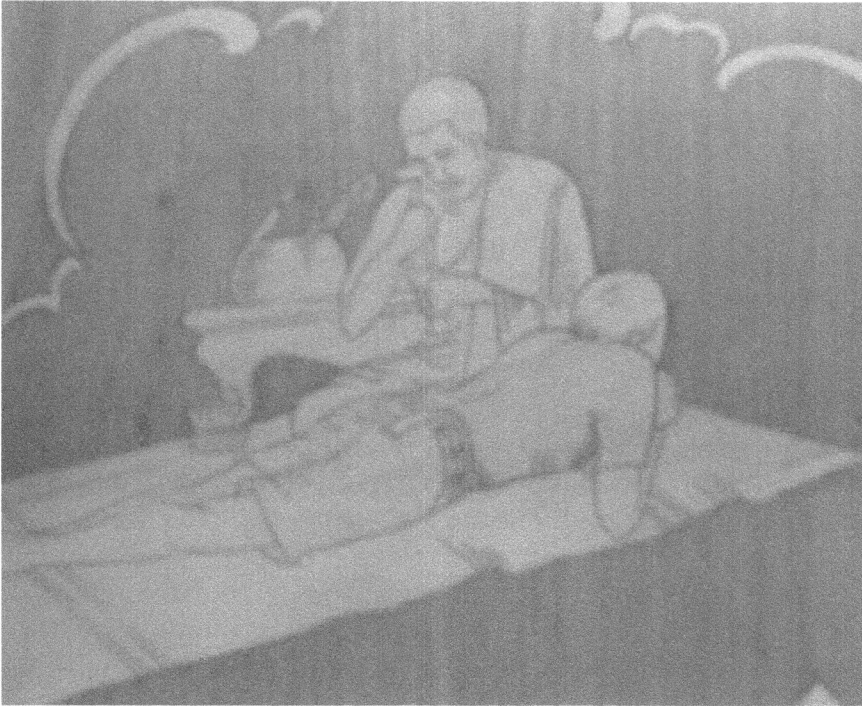

Traditional Thai Wood Cut Art of Monks practicing
Tapping with a wooden Hammer and point tool in
Wat, Amperwa, Thailand. Photo by author.

Use this work in an ethical fashion and with Common Sense!

Important... please read carefully!

Common sense would suggest that you wouldn't expect much in the way of negative side effects from SomaVeda® Bio-Tapp/ BET. This is because there are:

No surgical procedures.
No needles.
No pills or chemicals.
No pushing or pulling on the body.

Instead, there are just a few seemingly harmless procedures that involve tapping, humming, counting and rolling your eyes around in your head. By now, over several hundred thousand people have used similar and or related Tapping based techniques. The number of complaints are well under 1 percent. Once in awhile someone might report feeling a little achy, sore or nauseous. On occasion a few people report "feeling worse." Because these reports are so infrequent, it is unknown whether or not SomaVeda® Bio-Tapp/BET and/or derivative energy based techniques actually caused the problem. Some people, by the way, feel nauseous or "get worse" at the mere mention of their particular problem. They will do so whether or not SomaVeda® Bio-Tapp/BET is introduced. SomaVeda® Bio-Tapp/BET and related healing and balancing work are still in their beginning stages and we have much to learn.

It is possible that using SomaVeda® Bio-Tapp/BET could be deleterious to someone. Accordingly, you should assume that we are still in the experimental stage and use SomaVeda® Bio-Tapp/BET with appropriate caution.

Along these lines, I include below an important statement. It should be read carefully. Only go where you're invited. Stay only as long as necessary, do the minimum necessary, with the least side effects, and leave when appropriate! As we say in the Naturopathic community, "At the very least, Do no harm."

Others in the energy work world have said this before me and I'm sure many will say it after. We believe in common sense use and applications according to your actual ability, training and background. Most students and practitioner's will already understand what I have to say. The bottom line here is that we need to use common sense contraindications with SomaVeda® Bio-Tapp/BET and NOT apply it to people with serious issues UNLESS we have the appropriate training, experience, and an appropriate license if required or necessary to do so. It is truly exciting to discover a tool for healing so interesting and potentially profound. Yet, in good conscience, we must work from a cautious and skeptical frame of mind.

The issue is multi-faceted. One of the delightful aspects of SomaVeda® Bio-Tapp/BET (and its many cousins) is that, for the vast majority of people, it can be applied with little or no pain. Its gentle nature and non-invasive approach will finally provide a way for everyone to safely move towards wellness in mind, body, emotions and spirit. And why not? Why deny the public access to tools that are so often transformative on so many issues, and for most people, is gentle and easy to apply?

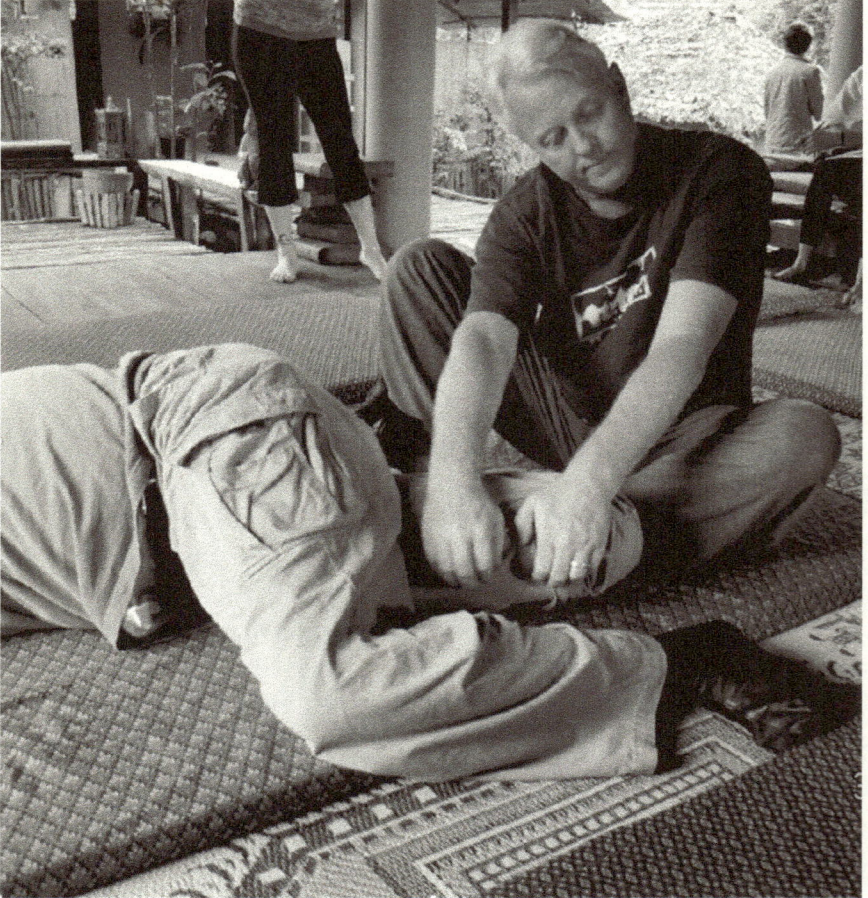

Aachan James demonstrates a SomaVeda® Indigenous, Traditional Thai Yoga side lying position in Pang Lang village, Thailand: November 2009

Common Uses For SomaVeda® Bio-Tapp/BET

Individuals who have not received the help and healing they previously thought the mainstream medical, psychological and or drug based industry would give them are finally able to take charge of their own healing process.

Yoga Therapists are integrating the practice in their sessions and routinely teaching the process to their clients for use at home.

Teachers are learning it for use with their students.

Coaches are learning it for use with their athletes.

Parents are learning it for use for themselves and with their children.

Physicians of all kinds are learning it for pain management with their patients.

Massage practitioners are blending it with their existing procedures for longer and more lasting results.

Spiritual leaders are applying it for their own issues and to those in need.

Chiropractors, acupuncturists and homeopathy practitioner's are augmenting their practices and teaching it to patients for self use.

Dealing with Side Effects

We don't know how many SomaVeda® Bio-Tapp/BET/EFT/ tapping enthusiasts are now using these procedures on behalf of others, but we could easily estimate that it exceeds 100,000's and has probably been applied over 1 million times worldwide. This wouldn't happen, of course, unless (1) substantial results were being received and (2) perceived dangers, or negative side effects, were minimal. While no experienced SomaVeda® Bio-Tapp/BET style practitioner can deny seeing substantial results, not everyone is aware that there CAN BE negative side effects, sometimes severe. Let me explain. Some people have been so badly traumatized and/ or abused in their lifetimes that they have developed severe psychological problems such as multiple personalities, paranoia, schizophrenia and other serious mental disorders.

While SomaVeda® Bio-Tapp/BET and its cousins have been helpful even in such severe cases, IN THESE INSTANCES IT SHOULD ONLY BE APPLIED BY A QUALIFIED PROFESSIONAL WITH EXPERIENCE IN THESE DISORDERS.

In no case can we recommend this or any treatment or therapy against the advice of a licensed physician. Any under the care of a Medical Doctor, Physician, or Psychiatrist must be recommended to consult with their physician before beginning any course of therapy. Why? First of all, because that's the law (common sense). Secondly, because some of these patients experience bad reactions whereby they go out of control. During healing crises it's possible that they could be harmful to themselves and others, and may need to be sedated or hospitalized. This is obviously no place for the novice, no matter how enthusiastic one might be with the tapping procedures.

Incidentally, we don't know yet whether tapping actually causes such side effects or bad reactions or if it is just the memory
of one's troublesome issues that precipitates such problems.
Nonetheless, if you have no experience in these areas, please
don't go where you don't belong.

How often do these bad reactions happen? In a psychiatric
care or hospital they are common. In everyday society they
are rare. In my own experience and in consulting with both my
own students and other professionals that have dealt with a
wide variety of emotional problems we have seen less than 1 in
1,000 clients have experienced such a severe abreaction. This
minimal percentage is given for perspective only. It is not to
suggest that SomaVeda® Bio-Tapp/BET practitioners should
"play the odds" and "go where they don't belong." On the
contrary, a novice SomaVeda® Bio-Tapp/BET or other
wholistic practitioner of any kind should use common sense
and NOT TRY TO ALLEVIATE or "CURE" AILMENTS THAT
ARE BEYOND THEIR CAPACITY OR TRAINING.

If you're in question or doubt as to your capacity to work with
a specific individual or specific condition or concern then refer
it out! Don't wing it. Again, I'm simply urging using a common
sense approach both for your safety and legality as a
practitioner and for the safety and integrity of your client.

However, with the aforementioned common sense
contraindications in mind, as the founder of the related EFT
technique, Gary Craig states, "Try it on everything!"

What are the issues with regard to practicing or
experimenting with SomaVeda® Bio-Tapp/BET on yourself
for your own personal issues? Well, you have every right and
authority to experiment and work on yourself without
necessity of having any external authority to give you
permission to do so.

Our Agreement

Accordingly, the following common sense statements constitute a legal agreement between us.

Please read these statements carefully; This material takes the form of a thorough discussion, explanation and demonstration of a very impressive personal improvement tool. It is not a training program in psychology or psychotherapy.

**Subject to the other provisions of this agreement, you may use SomaVeda® Bio-Tapp/BET on behalf of yourself or others.

** NAIC Inc., SomaVeda College of Natural Medicine: The Thai Yoga Center, Anthony B. James, Meta Journal Press, our authorized representatives and or teachers cannot and will not take responsibility for what you do with these techniques.

Accordingly...

**You are required to take complete responsibility for your own emotional and/or physical well being both during and after studying this material. **

You are also required to instruct others whom you help with SomaVeda® Bio-Tapp/BET or to whom you teach SomaVeda® Bio-Tapp/BET, to take complete responsibility for their emotional and/or physical well being at all times.

**You must agree to hold harmless anyone involved with SomaVeda® Bio-Tapp/BET from any claims made by anyone whom you seek to help with SomaVeda® Bio-Tapp/BET or to whom you teach SomaVeda® Bio-Tapp/BET.

**We urge you to use these techniques under the supervision of a qualified practitioner, therapist or physician. **

Don't use these techniques to try to solve a problem where your common sense would tell you it is not appropriate. If you do not agree with the foregoing, or cannot comply, please give notice and withdraw yourself from this training immediately. Otherwise, we have an agreement and we expect you to live by it.

What are "Bio-transformational Technologies"?

They are tools and technologies for adapting, re-organizing, balancing, healing, transforming and liberating the human biological machine.

We define people, ourselves, as stress adaptive, electro-biological organisms, i.e.. "machines." As such we are developed, shaped and "organized" by and according to various stressors.

What are the stressors that cause either healthy or unhealthy adaptation? These stressors are:

A) Stress built into the machine itself (tension or the machine's own internal resistance to simply being alive).

B) Stress from cultural programming (pressure to function, to conform or fit in, regardless of appropriateness or suitability for individual composition).

Acculturation is stressful in that normal familial and societal pressure takes into consideration little or nothing relating to the specific individuals design, makeup, personal limitations and strengths including those under personal inclinations.

Cultural programming is actually opposed to individual personal expression and treats all such as aberrations, even to the point of trying to isolate or destroy machines operating too far out of the norms.

This is especially true for individuals who elect to engage in activities designed to awaken and/or transform the personal machine.

These efforts make the body a more functional apparatus for transformation and expression of vital life energies and their corresponding positive emotional states such as love, compassion, equanimity and joy without bias or discrimination.

The stressors, when negative lend themselves to creating a state or condition or "Biopathy" with primary symptoms of "Sympatheticotonia."

What is Biopathy?

Biopathy is a contracture of the organisms Matrix and the TPB (Tangible Physical Body) emphasizing sympathetic nervous action dominance and activity i.e. "Sympatheticotonia."

What are the symptoms of Biopathy?

Psyche symptoms are negative fear, phobia, anxiety, general loss of conscious control of mind and emotions in a spiral of deterioration.

     a. Concentric movement and rigidity of physical and or postural attitude

     b. Stiffness, Inflexibility of mind and mental process

     c. Reflexive conditioning and progressive submission to negative and increasingly negative thoughts and thought patterns.

     d. Development of armoring and conditioned localized spasm forming both local areas of rigidity and corporately generalized loss of functions and circulation of life force, Prana, Chi, Orgone as well as actual circulation of vital substances of the body i.e. fluids, secretions, oxygen, lymphatic and a corresponding increase in edema, stagnation and proportional atrophy of first local area tissue, then general deterioration of the entire system.

     e. Energetically may be evidenced by imbalance and discord in the Matrix or energetic body seen as discord in Dosha, Chakra, Sen and Nadi. Hyper and or hypo sensitivity of Lom, points, Marma and lines, Nadi and or Thai Sen lines. Restrictions and inability to assume asana and distortions of asana in practice as well as in reduced ability to perform common and ordinary tasks.

Efforts to do just about anything within the normal course of life would be or seem to be more difficult. This difficulty could be mental, emotional or physical. This difficulty might or might not be accompanied by pain.

     f. Complex Symptomology: Symptoms can also be combined in the sense of the bioemotional, biophysical, biopsychic. Bioenergetic and biosexual manifestations may occur in either sequence or all at once in varying degree.

Our Developmental Plateau

Currently we have reached an evolutionary hiatus or plateau. Previously, there may have been some progress towards evolution of our species, however, up to this point it was mechanistic evolution. According to this system's way of thinking, we are still inherently no different than the progenitors of our species, the Neanderthal! The bulk of daily human life concerns and activities are basically the same. Security, survival, procreation, sex and so forth. Expression of ego and personality as primordial imperatives and so called inner expressions of love, communication, knowledge, art as secondary. You might say that some of the outward appearances or esthetics of life have changed, but have we as a species really changed?

For the last several thousands of years of biological time we have achieved a level of stagnation. Our cultures have modeled our average level of consciousness. Ideas and technologies for expressing our consciousness have not changed. For example, we still solve territorial disputes with yelling, pulling hair and swinging clubs. Only now we call yelling "Sophisticated Propaganda" and "spin." We call pulling hair "Elite surgical strike teams." We call clubs "Smart Bombs!"

Those among us who perpetuate the most extreme, most insane and most violent disturbances against the common good, peace and welfare of the populace are generally those claiming to be "Spiritual" and/or "Moral" authorities. Every conceivable, horrific act and offense possible to imagine, is carried out in the representation of "Moral" , "Ethical," "Spiritual" and "Legal" authority.

The truth is that the expression of these concepts is directly related to the transformation of the individual into levels of consciousness. We can say that each machines activity and expression of higher principles is relative to their level of evolution or Alchemy. For example, the concepts expressed as moral, ethical, spiritual and legal, in and of themselves, are not lower. However, when expressed and manifested by lower beings (relative state of transformation) they take on the quality of the lower consciousness.

In classical Alchemical terms, we speak of four states: Lead, Copper, Silver and Gold. Use them as metaphors for a relative state of transformation and level of consciousness. The expressions of "morals, ethics, spiritual and legal" of the lead alchemy person is formatory, mechanistic, unreasoned and violent. The same concepts expressed by a "Gold alchemy person are fair and intentional, reasoned, enlightened and liberated. By this same reasoning and illustration, those of the Copper and Silver Alchemy are being somewhere in between Gold and Lead on a continuum.

We believe the un-examined, un-transformed person is incapable of practically expressing these type of qualities in a consistent and intentional way.

The level of consciousness as expressed by the so called "Modern" world culture is exactly at the same level as that practiced by so called primitive culture. The words "primitive" and "modern" are meaningless when used in the context of levels of self realization and consciousness and/or transformational evolutionary process. Primitive simply states, "That was then" vs. the Moderns, "This is now." However, from the point of view of conscious, intentional evolutionary process, they are the same.

Our species, at some point, became locked into a loop of being and patriarchical mechanicality relatively early in our development as organic biological evolution. There are systems which attempt to express this idea for those who have access to them, such as Jnana Yoga (Vivekananda),

Self Realization teachings of Paramhansa Yogananda and the Gurdjief Enneagram teachings as well as the theories of Chakras in Ayurveda and Tantric Yoga for example. They show that in every path of occurrence and development there is clearly a point where ordinary processes cannot continue. They will hang, crystallize or loop one point where there must be stimulation or energy from outside in order for the process to continue, and another point where there must be a shift or change of state from within the process its self.

The main reason simply being that once we as a species achieved biological and numerical ascendancy and organic supremacy over most other life on the planet, there was no longer sufficient stress or the right kind of pressure to continue the process of evolution and transformation internally for the majority of the population. All subsequent development has been focused almost entirely on external power, control, comfort and life technology with rare exception.

28

The Two Kinds of Human Beings

I want to preface my following comments with the following statement. Nothing in what I am about to share is meant or intended to indicate genetic, race or sexual gender as a factor. The "two kinds of Human Beings" are metaphorical constructions to enable us to see ourselves, perhaps in a new or novel way. We are all, each and every one of us, both types inherently as every person has some of the baser qualities and the higher potentialities as well. I make this statement to clearly separate my comments and work from those Eugenics philosophies and psychological theories which espouse inequalities, or perceived differences as excuses for bad behaviors of unlimited variety and extent.

From as far back as back goes, there have been two distinctive kinds of human beings sharing this world. This revolutionary concept alone will explain much of the nature of our world and why things are as they are. These two kinds evolved at the same time, in the same conditions of life and share genetic material. However, they represent radically different and divergent biological expressions of humanity. The first kind, the most common kind, by orders of magnitude, is virtually entirely reactive and has a life almost entirely based on the cause and effect of external events and pressures. This first common type is characterized further by internal formatory reactive reasoning and justifications. The reactive reasoning and being accrues over time as this species goes through its limited life cycle. This first species comes in a few models easily recognizable to the trained observer.

The second kind, on first glance, looks to be very similar to its more numerous cousin. The evolutionary qualities for which it represents a leap of development are all electrical in nature vs. just biological. On the material plane, this second species has all of the same mechanical features, strengths and limitations as the first, however, it contains within its design the possibility of transforming its self under its own internal decision and will into a self realized conscious being with expanded faculties and cognitive processes, spanning multiple dimensions. We all have dimensions and unseen aspects of life outside of our common or ordinary purview. The second man may have a life not entirely defined nor limited by time and space as commonly considered and is aware of this! I mean by this the possible ability of carrying information and consciousness outside of the physical life and death of the machine. Just as the first Lung Fish represented the equivalent of a biological leap, as it was transitional between the water life and the life in the world of air and sun, this second or new man is a leap and transitional form between the physical and the electrical world of energy and fields and vital life essence which transcends multiple dimensional spectrums of the life equation.

Man #2, or the NEW MAN/WOMAN is invisible by direct observation to #1. Number one perceives its evolutionary and divergent cousin indirectly as an influence, effect or feeling, and is not wholly able to relate directly to the #2, but able to be influenced by #1. Man #1 will assume that #2 is essentially the same based on external appearances alone.

We believe there are #3's, 4's and so on, based on this same principle of indirect observation and influence..

The life and existence of #2's as a natural occurrence of universal principles, suggest this -- just as #1's perceive the existence of #2's by indirect effect, #2's by indirect effect and signs of influence infer the possible existence of #3's and #4's and so on. In other words we cannot see these other types as outwardly they appear very similar or exactly the same and share all the common body typing qualities and machine based variation the differences are in the internal lives and the way these new types create influence patterns of living and thought. They don't look different. They just are different.

#1's think and believe that we are all the same and share the same experiences and opportunity of life. #2's know this is not true!

Where does the New Man live or what is it's habitat? Well, it is inside the former of course! The New Man or New Woman is the new creation, intelligence, being and essence that manifest in the person as they awaken and become aware of their electrical, energetic and essential nature apart from the machine.

Any Man/Woman # 1 can become a #2 with repurposing of life focus, knowledge, self observation and effort or the right kind of work.

What kind of man or women is BET for?

SomaVeda® Bio-Tapp/BET is balancing for #2's. This is because the more awakened and newly evolving being and its electrical and multi-dimensional character requires special healing techniques. In the medicine for #1, we are primarily concerned with the integrity, function and structure of the machine, as well as number ones fuels, processes, effluents and metabolism. Additionally, we consider the "bugs," parasites, pests, toxins, temperature and even the weather that to which it is exposed. Maintain, keep or return these to acceptable norms, and the #1 kind is considered pretty much healthy. Mental, emotional and spiritual states are more of the reflexive, associative side of life. Generally speaking, if outside or external factors and functional operation of the machine are pleasant or favorable, the #1 experiences inner well being. #1 therapy and healing work is primarily about pain.

The #2 requires a different set of criteria for wellness, some of which is found in seeking stimulation which superficially might appear to be painful! This intentional seeking of pressure and first hand information is creating what we call "Voluntary Suffering." Whereas the #1 suffers it does so mechanically and perhaps with little conscious participation, the #2 must find that which makes it a bit uncomfortable to stimulate its electrical nature to literally produce inner friction and fire, which will in turn generate special frequencies of energy which is food for the soul or true essence.

The #2 desires inner alignment and inner harmonic concordance over and above the simple functionality of the machines in which its essence in life chooses to manifest. It looks for harmony states and equilibriums that may be quite subtle. The #2 at some point may elect to entirely disassociate from the limitations of the physical machine's life once it has served its primary functions as a **Stress Adaptive** *Human Biological Transformational Apparatus* (HBTA).

So, primary therapy for the #2 is less about the structure and functional operation of the machine, the pain experience of the machine, as it is about organizing energetic fields of influence to create harmonics and equilibriums conducive to multiple dimensional perceptions and expressions of consciousness.

A New Definition of Pain

We may still use common references such as pain. As a term "pain" for certain qualities of disharmony, imbalance or state of being, it is useful. However, in our proposed new way of understanding, real pain is represented as an impacting interference wave pattern which causes distortion fields in the Matrix Body and which do not support integration of the awakened consciousness. Simply stated, pain is a certain type or quality of disturbance or distortion of the electrical field of the body. The distortion fields manifest in the machine as negative emotions in all of their infinite diversity of expressions and intensity.

The negative emotions are complicating and contributing factors in every form of disease and imbalance of any persistent or chronic nature. There is no difference between so called chronic physical imbalance and chronic or persistent emotional or mental imbalance apart from the nefarious role of negative emotions. The negative emotions are the symptoms, of deeper electrical distortions.

Relating negative emotions and their diverse expressions as disturbances of the body's electrical fields gives rise to the "Discovery Statement" quoted so often by Gary Craig founder of EFT (Emotional Freedom Technique). The discovery statement is, **"The cause of all negative emotions is a disruption in the body's electrical system."**

Our understanding of what pain is says that "pain is the awareness of disruption of the electrical fields in the body, and experience of the negative emotions." The dominance of distortions and disruptions of the body's electrical fields and the greater deviation from harmonious and harmonic norms equals loss of functional states. If the body's mission, function and purpose in this life is to be a vehicle and/or HBTA then it is these distortions which provide the primary impediment. It is these distortion patterns and their harmonic aggregates and the negative emotion they spawn which keep the essence from achieving ascendency. These negative and dysfunctional states keep the machine completely and blindly in various nap like states or sleep. Although in the extreme, severe pain can sometimes act as a conscious shock. However, this is not a reliable way to awaken and as often as not will leave one heading for the Bardo in a confused and disoriented state of mind. (Bardo is an intermediate state of being described in the Tibetan Book of The Dead as existing between one life or existence and the next.)

We come together as an expression of affinity patterns because we share attention and frequency of consciousness. Or perhaps it is just because we have tried everything else and failed. You would not be drawn to this type of work and healing way unless you already have achieved certain levels of awareness and perception. This work is invisible to most sleep walkers, except in the rare exception when they might "notice" it. It is irritating! Even the idea of it can be irritating.

It is initially not received as "Balancing" or healing at all. It is as if, while you were in a very deep sleep, someone or something kept pricking you just enough to have you whine and move about, but not enough to wake you or for you to become aware of what was the matter.

This work is not for sleep walkers, at least not for those who are always asleep. It is for the newly awakened person.

The person who is suffering from the consequences of that awakening by now is being acutely aware of the imbalances evident in the machine, and now more than ever, sensitive to layers of distortion and the role and expressions of negative emotions in every area of life.

We have always been partners together in the eternal, which now exist as pure form in the realm of energy. We are together as partners working to solve the riddles of our common existence and manifestation in this material world. We are here together, by communion of our common purpose and union of our corporate energetic nature to overcome the limitations of our individual physical selves. We have help! We are help for one another and all together. One of the secrets of the #2 is that there may not be "many," there may only be one. Within that one is a continuum of expression and variation of frequency.

We work together because we have always worked together. We are each other's eternal Boddhisatva or liberating partners and fellow guides. We are our own benevolent deity, and we are each others Heruka (Tibetan Buddhist Wrathful Diety) and demons.

Our ambition is to be real and to know the whole story. What is our nightmare? To be less than real. To be fractured and alone. To be dark and empty . To be kept or held low and helpless before the afflictions inside and out against our will. Since we are Boddhisatva let us step forward and be guides in light and life touching, speaking, balancing, restoring, healing and unifying one another. Since we are Heruka, let us with great joy consume the unproductive and dead parts of our selves without care or mercy as these parts are NOT REAL!

In practice, we are attempting to release the bound up interference patterns and the harmonics of their aggregates, as well as the negative emotions entirely from which they originate. In a thousand ways, Quan Yin Boddhisatva reaches out with ten thousand lotus hands each representing one dance of liberation, one practical expression of perfected compassion, one technique for the manifestation of awakening and one step towards the great liberation of the boundless being and true essence.

One example is of the joy found in a place where pain is not the ruler, and standard of ones being, by which life is not defined and interpreted through or by the distorted spectacles of suffering in its infinite variety. Yes, the dance of liberation, to know that we are now and always have been the expression of our own perfected luminosity.

So, begin to work with this thought: "What is now before me is a reflection of my own perfect luminosity. Even though I have this manifestation of my negative emotions, I deeply and completely accept myself."

To be in this state is to be in a different place, a different realm of existence and life entirely. This work is Bardo work and when diligently applied will provide assistance and support for the journey.

How To Do A Basic SomaVeda® Bio-Tapp/BET Session

Perhaps it is a bit challenging to attempt to describe the "why" and "how" Bio-Tapp/BET works in words. However, to actually do the method is very simple. For some too simple! One of the only criticisms we have received or challenges to it as a healing methodology is that it on appearance is simple, on the verge of even appearing silly. For this reason especially, I have attempted to go into some detail on possible ideas, theories and explanations as to why something so simple and silly should be considered rational and possibly profound.

The Bio-Tapp/BET technique can be brought into play at any time during any session as negative emotions or energy disruptions may manifest. The basic technique can be done as a stand alone session. It can be done before, during or after a session in an integrated fashion. This is highly recommended as the full SomaVeda®program will balance many different issues and aspects for the client and create a nurturing and loving environment. A loving environment is a more trusting environment. This BET protocol can also be done as an adjunct and/ or non-locally, over the phone for example. We also recommend that you teach it to your client for home use.

Emphasize that the client is always in control and responsible for their well-being at all times during this process. It can be stopped or adjusted at any time. You might actually say, or use the words, "Taking responsibility for your own welfare and comfort," or something along those lines.

1. Determine the primary complaint or issue. Try to be as specific as possible. Be alert for underlying issues which might be more fundamental.

2. Ask for or generate an index number for severity of current state or pain. This should be a number between zero and ten with zero being little or no symptom and ten being more than they can bear or severely acute.

3. Start with light rubbing of the Setup Point for Psychological Reversal ("Sore Point" or "Karate Chop Point') and recite the organizing statement;

"Even though I have this_____, I deeply and completely accept myself." 3X (You can adjust or change this statement to better suit yourself or client.)
> Do the Basic Algorithm
> Do the Hand Points Algorithm
> Do the Nine Gamut Set Algorithm

4. Reassess and see if the index number has improved. If the complaint is resolved either you're done or move on to another issue. If the primary complaint is not resolved or if another complaint or issue has surfaced in it's place, then go back and repeat Steps #2, #3 and #4... Perhaps substituting the words "Even though I still have this _____ I deeply and completely accept myself."

5. Repeat as often as necessary.

(Advanced practice could also include testing for Psychological Reversal, Energy Allergies and Toxins, etc.)

Initial Points for Basic SomaVeda®
Bio-Tapp/BET Treatment Algorithm

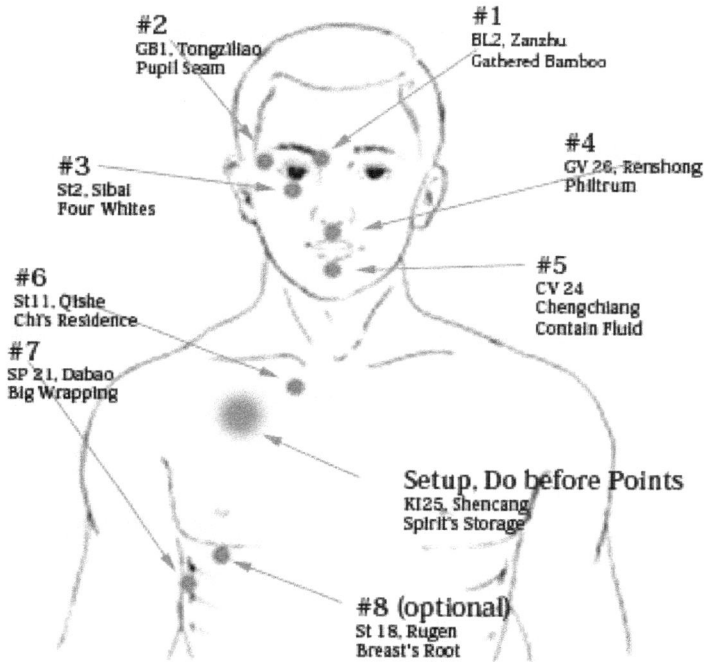

#2
GB1, Tongziliao
Pupil Seam

#1
BL2, Zanzhu
Gathered Bamboo

#3
St2, Sibai
Four Whites

#4
GV 26, Renshong
Philtrum

#6
St11, Qishe
Chi's Residence

#5
CV 24
Chengchiang
Contain Fluid

#7
SP 21, Dabao
Big Wrapping

Setup, Do before Points
KI25, Shencang
Spirit's Storage

#8 (optional)
St 18, Rugen
Breast's Root

1) Over the Eye (OE)
2) Beside the Eye (BE)
3) Under the Eye (UE)
4) Under the Nose (UN)
5) Under Mouth (UM)
6) Collar Bone (CB)
7) Side of Body (SB)

Setup Point for Psychological Reversal (See "Sore Point" or "Karate Chop Point")

Hand Points for Basic SomaVeda®
Bio-Tapp/BET Treatment Algorithm

1) Side of Thumb
2) Side of Index finger
3) Side of middle finger
4) Side of little finger
5) 9 Gamut Point on Back of Hand
     (Halfway between 4th and 5th metacarpal)
6) Half way on side of hand (Karate Chop)

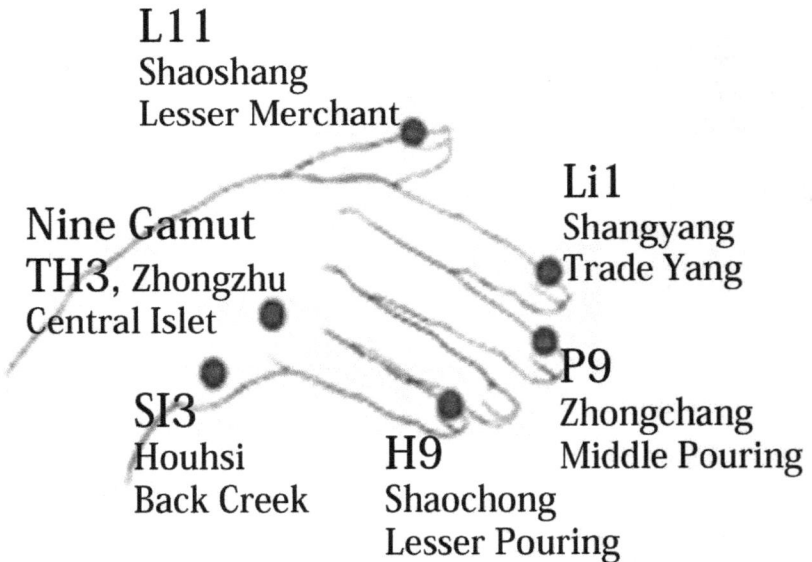

L11
Shaoshang
Lesser Merchant

Li1
Shangyang
Trade Yang

Nine Gamut

TH3, Zhongzhu

Central Islet

P9
Zhongchang
Middle Pouring

SI3
Houhsi
Back Creek

H9
Shaochong
Lesser Pouring

Nine Gamut Set for
Basic SomaVeda® Bio-Tapp/BET Treatment Algorithm

A) Start tapping 9 Gamut point and recite organizing statement "Even though I have this_____, I deeply and completely accept myself." 3X

B)
    1) Close Eyes
    2) Eyes Hard Down Right
    3) Eyes Hard Down Left
    4) Look up and around Left to Right
    5) Look up and around Right to Left
    6) Hum a song (Happy B'day)
    7) Count to Five
    8) Hum a song (Happy B'day)

Discovery Statement:
    The Cause of ALL negative emotions is disruption of the body's energy system.

The Thirty Four SomaVeda®
Bio-Tapp/BET Premises

Premise #1: Everything is Energy:

We are construed of 2 primary interacting infringing electric fields and corresponding interference patterns, and harmonics as expressed in modulated wave forms and frequency of light. One field we call higher and equate with the essential being, spirit, conscience or Atman/Soul. One we call lower which is the sum of our organic manifestation and consciousness of the body, also known as "The Machine." The lower is the primary and greater influence in undeveloped man and woman and is the vehicle which carries, nurtures and has potential to transform the higher. The lower transformational characteristics are nonfunctional until they are intentionally triggered under special circumstances with specific access methods. Because it is the machines nature to function as a transformational apparatus, it will occasionally lend itself to moments of higher activity, either randomly or as a result of external stimulation.

However, these periods of more correct or higher functioning are not sustainable or even predictable. It could be seen like a high performance race car with a novice driver. The car could perform well and drive very fast with exceptional handling characteristics in its proper context with a professional driver, perhaps in a specific environment and track. However, under the guidance of the novice, untrained or inexperienced driver it barely limps along, occasionally spurting into a faster speed or slamming the brakes on as the driver is overcome with fear, feeling that the vehicle is not really controllable! Such is the relationship of our higher to lower. Further complicated is that our machine is a self evolving, self training mechanism with its own limited awareness completely able to "drive" without a driver!

Premise #2: Everything is Connected to Everything Else on some level:

These fields of interacting infringing electrical energy exist in the wider domain of the greater living field of all organic life, the world. As the native Americans say, "Mitakueous Oyasin," meaning we are all related. This is also a restatement of the Hermetic and Alchemical statement of "As above, As below."

We as energy and consciousness manifesting as a human biological machine are a representation of the higher and lower cosmologies which form the greater cosmos of our existence. The only difference between our internal energetic, atomic, or quantum mechanisms and those of our solar system is one of scale. The same principle extends to the world of the Microcosm and microscopic to beyond the sub-atomic.

In certain Oriental traditions, Chinese Taoism for example, the first trigram of the "I Ching" (Chinese Book of Changes) is three bars representing "Heaven, Man, Earth." What's more interesting is that not only do we mirror in function and action the principles of these higher and lower cosmologies, but that it is two way (if two is virtually infinite!). These cosmos are affected by us as well. Astrological systems are either attempts at quantifying the interrelation of these cosmos and fields of influence, or as metaphor's for discerning internal relation-ships and states occurring within us and in our perceptions of our environment. In Quantum Physics, the idea or mathematical statement that describes this inter connection is called "Entanglement." Entanglement Theory postulates that at the smallest level of matter and energy literally everything is connected to everything else.

Premise #3: We are part of everything:

The World exists in the context of the greater fields of the solar system and universe at large.

Premise #4: Everything affects everything else:

All of these fields impact and influence one another causing patterns of influence and distortion. These patterns of overlapping fields cause secondary and tertiary distortions called harmonics and resonance.

Premise #5: We are Stress Adaptive Electrical-Biological Organisms:

Stress equals energy. Stress adaptation is how we are influenced (distorted/ shaped)by the energies and influences we exist in and are part of. Organic tissue is a sum representative of electrical fields with specific frequencies and corresponding harmonics creating distinctive wave forms. The life, operation and shape, the function and all possible actions of the tissue reflect these expressed distinctive wave forms. This includes both functional and dysfunctional adaptation. Knowing how we are shaped by stress opens the door to intentionally shaping stress to give us the adaptations and healthy functions we seek.

Premise #6: Greater fields influence lessor fields:

The various forms of consciousness and attention represent possible overtones and fields of influence which can alter the shape and frequency of the inferior wave forms.

Premise #7: The shape and function of the tissue is determined by the wave form it models:

The shape and function of the tissue is determined by the wave form it models in local spacetime and is a dynamic changeable equilibrium. The interaction of all tissues working together may be modelled in the same manner as a mathematical equation of harmonics and distortion or impacting and overlapping relevancies.

Premise #8: Attitudes are like wires, which connect us to events:

Attitudes = Electrical fields which are generative consciousness. Attitudes are that which creates harmonics and subsequent fields of lesser or minor influence. Wires = Harmonics i.e. secondary and tertiary subsequently occurring electrical fields, distortions and probabilities resulting from the interaction and influence of the primary fields or attitudes. Events = The material manifestation of the preceding electrical fields and their subsequent harmonics, i.e. organic material and structure of the body corpus and actual manifestations which occur around the body as well.

To change the events (i.e. the tissue state in local time/space equilibrium) *to which we are subject* (which are the end result subjectively of our own electrical fields and the corresponding distortions, shapes and functions those fields organize and generate) *We must first change our attitudes.* We must change the covalence, frequency, amplitude and shape of the fundamental electrical potential and the associated wave forms and harmonics which these potentials and wave forms represent.

Although these fields have a life outside of the perceived limitations of time and space, we can affect fundamental changes in the wave forms with a cause and effect set of intentional impingements on local distortions. We create this balancing by bringing attention, intention, consciousness/ awareness, energy, breath and pressure to bear on specific local of distortion.

Energy precedes consciousness. Consciousness precedes attention. Attention precedes Intention. Intention precedes application of discipline and the possible alteration of manifestation according to conscious design. Whether intentional, conscious or not, energy precedes physiology.

Premise #9: Every event or occurrence experienced throughout life is recorded or stored:

Every event or occurrence experienced throughout life is recorded or stored as a local distortion of the matrix body/mind continuum based on affinity principle. Affinity principle is basically similar to the "Law of Similars" in alchemy and homeopathy. Like attracts like. Memory stored as local distortion fields, attracts similar occurrences and layer them in specific local according to similarity or perception of similarity.

Every subsequent or similar event or occurrence is stored in the same way in the same place regardless of whether the events or occurrences were actually the same. These points may accumulate layers of energy (overlapping but slightly dissimilar wave forms) virtually without limitation. These specific locale may be measured inferentially as areas of higher neurologic and electrical activity. The cumulative effect of these aggregates of overlapping distortion wave fields (memories and impressions) may be taken as an example of Karma.

Premise #10: It takes energy to store and to preserve information:

It takes energy to store and to preserve these referenced local distortion fields. More distortion or overlapping disharmonic (negative/maladaptive/disruptive) wave forms in a specific location require more energy. Fewer overlapping distortion wave fields in a specific locale equal more energy (information) available to the machine.

The energy (information) stored in these distortion fields is not available as a general resources for the rest of you. Where is your energy being used? How much of your energy is being used to store and preserve old issues and negative emotional constructs? How much information about yourself is not available because it is tied up, allocated energetically to maintaining these distortion fields. Information is just another word for energy. The truth will set you free. Truth is information. Information is energy. Energy will set you free, but not just any kind of energy.

Premise #11: It takes energy to make energy:

It takes energy to make energy! By reducing disequilibriums as represented by the distortion and accumulative wave patterns or aggregates, energy (electrical, magnetic) is returned to the use and allocation of the machine. It is returned to the greater field, the "Magnum Energeticum" to the "One." This strengthens and amplifies the greater fields helping to increase its overriding, generative and controlling action. Less distortion in the general field means stronger resonance and primary manifestation of the super consciousness seeking to manifest.

It takes energy to make energy! Actually, this is a misstatement. What I mean is that we do not actually create energy, because that is not possible! What we do is affect, manage, transform and change the state of energy. We have a finite quantity of energy available to us in various forms at any given time. Finite means that it is in some way limited. Our energy reserve has been up to this point allocated in an unconscious and mechanical or formatory fashion as dictated by biological and situational necessity. The goal is now to create conditions whereby a thoughtful individual may reallocate these energy reserves towards more balanced and productive use.

Premise #12: Negative interference patterns are not real:

Not real in the sense of being original or fundamental causes of disruptions. The negative minor wave interference patterns are essentially symptoms of other more basic disruptions of the bodies energy system. They are negative and have no real life or generative capacity above what they steal or poach or divert from the primary.

Let's use Harbor porpoise as a metaphor for this principle. You will often see these dolphins surfing in and around large vessels as they move around the channels and waterways in which these porpoise live. They find a large boat moving in the water which is creating a "Wake," or bow wave.

They opportunistically present themselves to the bow wave of the vessel, the low pressure area of the wave, where they are picked up and pushed forward. As long as the vessel maintains adequate speed (pressure potential), the porpoise can persist and "ride the wave" without much effort. They do not make the wave. They do not generate, store or cause the energy that the wave manifest or represents. They are not reflective of the consciousness that the boat, captain and crew represent. For example, the boat was not designed as a vehicle or transport for the porpoise.

The porpoise' consciousness and life in the wake, or the wave in front of the boat in no way reflects the "Higher" consciousness and energy of the captain. The porpoise represent a probability of occurrence. In this example the porpoise are basically harmless probabilities occurring in the life and function of the vessel. They represent little in the way of danger or disturbance for the mission, function and purpose or life of the vessel and crew.

But what if there were so many of the porpoise, or more of another species such as whales, or they were all so large that the boat had to adapt to their presence? What if the vessel in our metaphor was forced to change course or maneuver around them? What if the necessity of adapting to the interference or these creatures impeded the vessel?

To change the relationship of the porpoise interference to the boat, all the Captain would have to do is to slow down and or change direction or both. The Dolphins would then simply dissapate or disperse and then would no longer be able to "interfere" with the boats progress.

This is a simplified way of seeing a negative potential for accumulated overlapping impingement wave forms in specific locale. Do not take the metaphor too literally, because we love porpoises! We call these points or locale Lom, Wind gates, Chakra, pressure points, trigger points, areas of high neurologic energy.

Premise #13: Reduce the many equals increase the one:

One goal or objective is to reduce interference patterns and the loss of vital energy and integrity that they represent. We want to increase and to restore full vitality and energy to the machine in order that the machine be fully supported as a Bio-Neuro-electrical transformational apparatus. Layered interference patterns are the "fractured self" which the ancients were referring to. To not be fractured and split is to be whole – to be one. This is also the true meaning of "integrity."

How can we be true? How can we exemplify qualities of oneness and integrity when what we call I is effectively the aggregate of literally thousands upon thousands of layered interference wave forms and fields creating fractured, negative and unpredictable, unreliable manifestations which look like ego, which look like fear and inhibitions contrary to positive expression of life fore? Fractured, broken and disabled is not the platform from which to enable us to become our real selves according to our real nature, which is found in unity. Less fractured equals more "One-Like." Less fractured equals less "Ego-Like." Less fractured equals more energetic and capable-like.

Premise #14: Accumulated negative wave forms are karma:

The essence, soul or spirit is an electrical potential seeking to manifest in the greater field of organic life. Over a period of time, its ability to manifest clearly and with integrity is corrupted. The Buddhists call this process the manifestation of ego. Ego is the sum of local specific negative wave form impingement on the Matrix-Body-Mind continuum. Ego represents the sum of all aggregate disturbances and distortions accumulated over millions of years and life times. This is another definition of "karma."

By reducing and or eliminating these local field distortions and the corresponding aggregates of multiple overlapping impingements, we reduce chaos. We reduce misappropriation of vital energetic resources. We reduce mental, physical, emotional and spiritual distortions and imbalances as they are the result of distorted wave forms. Since removing or correcting/balancing any local disturbance field affects all of the local pattern disturbances and their harmonics in and near that local, it is possible to resolve hundreds, thousands, perhaps even millions of "Event Centered" impingement and negative wave forms or the Bad Karma of many lifetimes.

This is the mechanism giving the foundation of the concept of an individual possibly becoming enlightened in a single lifetime! Keep in mind, we cannot readily see these impingements and negative wave forms, aggregates, harmonics, and more within ourselves as they are "Natural" to us, like the forest to the trees kind of thing. This means the possibility of balancing them must, of necessity, require outside intervention or "Help." This is our true Achilles Heel. Our "Humility Clause" as fields are affected by other fields.

We need another individual or group of individuals to model the higher and more balanced state. So Karma is the accumulated effect and manifestation of negative wave forms accumulated and layered in specific locale over time. Any negative thought, action, deed or event can generate the negative wave form. As we said before, the field of the wave forms cluster or accumulate in specific locale based on affinity principle.

Reduction or elimination of the "Bad" Karma for a long complex path of life in a sleeping machine is perhaps not possible. However, it is possible to correct, balance and undo the Karma of specific identifiable local or points. Balancing even one point or the issue it represents affects the whole in a positive way. However, in the short term "balancing" can look odd as even a positive push into equilibrium and less disruptive wave forms is unsettling to the machine. Even therapy and correction is stressful! This is why we need help, guidance and support from knowledgeable persons to work through the unsteady periods towards real stability and pro-gress. Eventually when enough "Trees" are eliminated, we can do for ourselves, but for most this is just wishful thinking.

Premise #15: Be What You Know:

By definition, enlightenment or self realized, self consciousness is the result of removing the obscuring anomalies and the negative wave forms they represent.

Since these electrical nodes of accumulated negative energy themselves create further impacting waves and distortions of electrical potential, these potentials according to affinity principle are experienced as thoughts, actions, deeds, feelings, emotions and events both internal and external.

How can we be real, be one in the presence and overwhelming influence of so much stored dissonance? We cannot! We must use every tool at our disposal to reduce, balance and or eliminate these distortions to our fields of consciousness and being! To paraphrase the Buddha, "We must make our way to the portals that give upon liberty, and in every moment it is in our power so to do. That door is free of all bolts and bars save those that man himself has made."

"We must make our way," is the process of submitting to education and balancing therapy. The barriers to liberty are the obscuring anomalies of negative wave forms and their aggregates and harmonics. The door is the possibility and potential that exist when the limitations and energy waste common to unconscious, unexamined and unbalanced life is reduced and/or eliminated returning full access to energetic potential.

Freedom is not the end result but the beginning of what is possible when a correct and balanced man or woman begins to work on themselves and each other without pain, suffering, fear and all other similar negative expressions and manifestations.

Bolts and Bars are the unreal, negative, imaginary attitudes which drive us to and keep us in mechanical, sleeping and unconscious life. Enlightenment is not just knowing the state of how things are, but the being and doing based on putting the principles into daily work and effort. Be what you know.

Premise #16: Reducing Harmful External and Internal Interferences supports the Work:

How can we create a suitable Bio-Neuro Electrical foundation for work? How can we create opportunity for work? How can we support creation as principle of life? We do not awaken the sleeper within so much as we actually create a new person entirely. This is what was originally meant by being "Born Again." However, it is not outside agency or powers which awaken us. It is we who create and birth the new being, the new life essence.

Become a student, and then as a student volunteer. Once you volunteer follow the directions through until the exercise or project is complete. Notice how eager you are at the beginning and how very much you lose interest or get lazy before completing. Still, volunteer. To be a student means to be always ready to volunteer and to follow directions. Anything else is a tramp feature. Generate external and internal alignments which support balance and reduce waste and harm to the machine.

The following are some examples for reducing interferences. We divide this kind of work into either Externally focused or Internally focused efforts. Externally means to work or make disciplined efforts from the outside in. This covers externally focused self work. Working from the outside in includes, doing point work, and hands on, show humility by receiving conversation, even if not entirely comfortable, but with intention. If entirely comfortable, try not to fall asleep. Observe the machine, yourself, when receiving work and therapy. However, observe without judgment and associative thinking as much as possible. There is opportunity to see aspects and alignments, and affinities, which are normally not visible.

Engage in and practice an external focus discipline such as Yoga, dancing, theatre, art, martial arts or music. Learn to play a musical instrument for example.

Develop humility by practicing receiving.

Learn about and engage proper diet and supplementation/ nutrition. Feed the machine. Many disturbances to your energy can easily or completely be remedied by proper nutrition. Food is important. Kind and quality of food is important. Learn to recognize "Real Food" from imaginary, fantasy, nonfood materials which through careful manufacture and deliberate deception are marketed as Real Food. Avoid eating anything which has empty or NO identifiable nutritional value. Avoid chemicals made to appear as food. Avoid genetically modified or Hybrid "Almost" foods. As the machine does not recognize these things and reacts to them as intrusive events creating wave patterns which look like allergies and weaknesses.

A primarily plant based diet reduces the possibility and severity of many, many diet and or nutritionally related diseases and disorders. Maintaining a plant based diet on a daily basis is the easiest and most direct way to stimulate and support your immune system. It will likely reduce food born toxins, chemicals, plasticisers, pesticides and harmful bacteria which would otherwise be typical in a meat based diet. This kind of diet supports optimal weight, blood pressure and metabolism for all life activities. It invigorates and will increase sexual vitality as well in both men and women.

A plant based diet reduces stress for the individual, the community and the world. Meat production causes everything from the development and spread of diseases to deforestation and contributes to Global Warming! It supports wholesale mistreatment and abuse of both animals and ecosystems. All of which eventually come back to cause individual stress.

Good nutrition reduces harm from inside and outside. Simply reducing the short and long term affects of poor nutrition will allow you more energy and a better platform from which to work on perhaps more important issues. Your inner issues.

Consider toxicity and Deficiency. Try to reduce environmental interferences to the machine. This includes what the Chinese call External Pernicious Influences in Traditional Chinese medicine. These harmful or disruptive influences can be organic such as bacteria and viruses, pest and harmful organisms such as amoeba, liver flukes, and worms. They can be elemental such as too much of any natural force such as sun, wind, cold and water. They can be man made chemicals and pesticides as well as radiative, both nuclear waste and by products to ELF and EMF radiation. Extremely low Frequency such as from Sanguine or Military Over the Horizon Radar, Microwave and Electrical interference from High Voltage Power Lines and other more mundane producers of electrical radiation such as Cell Phones.

Spend time working outdoors in a natural environment. The unpolluted, oxygen enriched environment not only is less toxic to your machine, it is stimulating to all of the centers. Working close to the ground exposes you to the Earth's background magnetic field, one of the greater fields we are always seeking equilibrium with naturally.

This magnetic field is in itself balancing and has a tendency to reduce stress internally and externally. Of course, don't over work, and avoid over exposure. There is such a thing as over exposure to the natural elements.

Keep hydrated with good water and micro-nutrients and electrolytes. Salt water internally and on the surface of the skin conducts micro-currents of electromagnetic fields and currents. De-hydration is a factor in many forms of illness and imbalance. It defeats the proper functioning of the immune system and is a factor in edema and metabolism in the body. It's not enough to just have water. We need to make sure we have a sustainable source of micro-nutrients such as Trace Minerals to furnish all cofactor's necessary for optimal health. This includes all 92 trace minerals including 200 mcg. of Selenium for example to target and reduce potential and actual cancer risk.

Internally means to work or make disciplined efforts from the inside out. Practice exercises and meditations if you will to promote observation and will of attention. These can be anything which achieve the result, whether considered traditional or not. We are in a unique time in history where we have an opportunity to literally invent exercises without being bound by dogma of outmoded systems.

However, there is a caveat. Exercises and the states they engender must still be qualified against the measuring stick of what is productive and useful; otherwise it could just be glamour and entertainment locking us into sleep, negativity and imbalanced patterns. Prana Yama and Kriya Yoga are good examples of possibly effective work; however, these should only be practised under competent instruction as they also can cause harm or imbalance if not performed correctly. These types of exercise can help to coordinate and tie in external work with internal.

All exercises and activities are to create or support specific states of mind, which represent electrical fields, harmonics and sub-harmonics conducive to the right operation of the machine. The physical balancing is specifically to reduce the impingement of negative wave form aggregates locale. These aggregates appear in practical terms as negative states of mind, conflict and dissonant thinking, negative emotions and the expressions of negative emotions such phobia's, nightmares and various unproductive fixations and emotional vexations. All together we could call them the residuals of Karma.

Work occurs from all angles simultaneously towards the center. The center is a clear and unobstructed field of influence called the waking mind in partnership with a balanced machine. More simply than this we could say that the center we work for is a waking state free of the expressions of unreal negativity that includes negative attitudes, emotions, phobic states and all of their physiological counterparts.

These negative attitudes, emotions, phobic states and their physiologic, biochemical results are basically what we observe as common ailments, disease processes and mental weaknesses and illnesses. Even many so called "structural" or "traumatic" challenges and health problems still occur in the same way as eventual adaptations to preexisting anomalous and dissonant states of being. For example, many trauma occur as a result of accidents. Yes? Many of these accidents are considered to be avoidable. So, why were they not avoided? Why did we not see, stop, or slow down when it would have been prudent?

Much emotional trauma for example is interpersonal. What keeps us from being able to be communicative, compassionate and diplomatic that we are mean? Or what crafts the abusive personality? Many illnesses are caused or related to long term malnutrition, why do we not simply acknowledge this and make nutrition a basic part of every person's education?

More than this why do we not follow the sensible proscriptions and take the supplements, eat the quality food, drink the good water, etc? There is no end to this line of questioning, however, the answer is still pretty simple –

expedience and the nominal functioning of mechanical persons who, if nothing else, are masters of "Going with the flow."

The problem is that the flow of nominal human consciousness is leading us towards precipice of pain and suffering in every way conceivable. To wake up and move against the tide has to be the hardest work any of us will ever conceive or do and many will not be successful.

The forces and pressures to encourage us to follow the sleepy norm are enormous and to resist them we need help. Help comes in the form of flesh and blood persons – teachers, schools and communities – working in cooperation to become significant, and maybe to eventually be able to change something critical in a good way, and in a way that will endure.

Premise #17: We are working for the past, the now and the future:

We are working for the past, the now and the future. By working in this fashion we hope to reconcile and harmonize the effects of past discord and trauma in order to have a direct impact on reducing unnecessary suffering in the present time.

The origin of virtually all current negative emotional symptoms and energy imbalance is in the past. Modern Quantum Physicist have the theory that time , linear time as most people know it does not exist. That in fact it is an illusion or misconception based on a limitation of viewpoint. The past, present and future are concurrent variations of perception of the NOW. The universe is not really "past, present and future" it simply is. We understand this to mean in our own lives the past and the effects originating in the past are concurrent in some way with our current perception of now. We also understand that our future is concurrent as well.

By changing, releasing, balancing the disruptions of energy originating in the past experience we cause real time changes to our current condition. We are different now! By being different now we are also creating the template of possibility of being entirely different in the future at the same moment. Our future self is concurrent. Our future self is here now.

The Metta Sutra of Buddha Dharma Mantra reflects a similar understanding when it so clearly states "May I no longer participate in the origination cycle of the creation of suffering for myself or for other."

This statement may also be seen as referring to the principle of Karma. However, to no longer participate in the creation cycle of suffering requires one to be different entirely. To be different entirely means we have to undo those karmic bounds, the patterns of imbalance which form the basis of our existing self and state of being.

By literally time travelling to unwind cords of disharmony in the past we lighten the load we are dealing with in the present now, the right now.

Working from past issues is necessary to be in the present moment with out the burden of accumulated trauma that unresolved issues place on us every moment. By working in the now, we avoid recreating, regenerating and causing the same types of harm and issues that were visited upon us in and from the past.

We hope to create something that will persist even possibly after the physical death of the machine. "Native American cultures speak of working for seven generations." We are in the Bardo now, so to speak, and wish to make further progress in our life and afterlife. This could also be a metaphor for the present existence. Seven generations could be taken as seven Chakra cycles, seven Saturn returns, seven ages of man, etc.

Premise #18: The work continues after you die:

We cannot be certain of the actual progress of our partners in and during their life and practice. We acknowledge that there may be a period of instability immediately following the death of the machine. We will endeavor and make reasonable efforts to support our partners and others with post passing balancing by way of readings and recitation of the Bardo Thodol or guide book for the newly deceased.

This guide book is traditionally known as The Tibetan Book of the Dead.

I am saying many things here. One is that, YES it is possible to affect the energy of the newly deceased in a positive way. We are still connected for a short time, and if one is paying attention there is an opportunity to do something significant. I do mean this literally.

We also say for the purposes of argument that the Bardo State is also a metaphor for the here and now. We are in the Bardo now in this life. The problem is that we don't know it. If one of the prerequisites for getting through the Bardo is the recitation and acknowledgement of specific mantra which clearly demonstrate specific and required states of being, then the time to look for them is not after you're dead! Think "I do for you as I do for myself," i.e. your progress is also my progress. As in Premise 18, we may figuratively die many times in this current manifestation of life and something of substance may continue from figurative re-birth to re-birth.

Even if you don't believe in the Bardo or "life after death," then at least have in mind the idea of Karma or cause and effect principle in life. If we can agree that much of what we have to deal with today actually is derived from thoughts, actions, deeds in the past and we see ourselves as part of that process then everything we can do in the moment to break, refocus, redirect harmful energies however they manifest will have a beneficial effect on the future.

This beneficial effect, like the ripple in a pond, expands much beyond the apparent boundaries of our life.

If you just take past, present and future states of being as consecutive states that one would experience all together in one or this present life the end result is the same.

Premise #19: Advanced teaching includes study of symbols:

Advanced teaching includes study of symbols and art, icons and myth as they are metaphors for electrical field states and harmonics as experienced by the human essence or spirit in transition. Ayurveda Yantra such as the symbols for the Chakra, Tibetan Mandala, the Bardo Thodal (Tibetan Book of the Dead) and similar works of known and unknown origin are gold mines for such insight and information. Additionally great art from any generation can have similar effects. Symbols, art and icons have the capacity to reach past the nappy gate keepers and effect and stimulate changes in the deeper parts of us – parts not normally under our conscious control or awareness. The use of metaphors speaks to us without engaging the lower parts of the intellectual, emotional centers.

Premise #20: We chose to live and be this experience:

We chose to manifest in this world of existence to gain the possibility of this experience of life. We are here to work and we are not working alone. I also like to say, if there is such a thing as a corporate consciousness, one of the caveats we agreed upon before manifesting was that "No One Gets Out, Until Every One Gets Out"! Avatar, Reishi, Rinpoche, Buddha,

Boddhisatva, Transfigured Jesus after the cross, Illuminati all beg the question – Why come back? To work so hard and long to be free of the bonds of earth, mechanicality and the burdens of Karma and Ego, to then Post-transition and transfiguring ascension to then turn about and come back? Universally, to do what? To help us? Again I ask, why? A work premise is that this is hypothetical at best, because only the ascendant transfigured being could rightly say for sure, but the practical answer is that if in fact they come back its because they have to!

Our collective consciousness is bound together via the shared electrical fields that generate them in the first place. When the Tibetan Buddhist pray for the freedom of suffering and eventual enlightenment of all living beings, they really mean it. No one prays for this more than the reincarnated Boddhisatva and Rinpoches who know the true conditions of freedom, that no one is truly free until everyone is free!

If you knew this or believed this simple truth in your bones, would you live act, think or be any different? You would if you could. But that brings us back to "Doing." So in all honesty, we don't do because we are limited by not being able to do. Freedom is for those who can do. This system is, therefore, as much about freedom as anything else on a practical level.

Premise #21: The Matrix Body holds the Key to the Invisible world.

Energy based theories such as Chakra, Sen and Meridian, Nadi, Marma, Lom, Wind gate and corresponding psychology are hypothetical models for how the Chronic or Chief Negative Features manifest in a given person. The interaction between the Matrix Body and the Tangible Physical Body interacting and adapting to our life environment creates the "Ego" effect , personality constructs and the like.

Most of the time except in rare circumstances these separate personalities manifesting the ego are invisible to us. They are hidden to us. However, we have been given literal road maps describing the hidden features in order to allow us to better work and understand ourselves and others.

Premise #22: We are fundamentally, literally energy.

A human being is an energy or electrical field within the larger energy or electrical field called biological life. Quantum physics gives us the idea that there is actually nothing that is not entirely made up of energy. If energy is all there is, then as part of "all that there is," we are energy too.

Premise #23: All is God, All is Energy, All is Electrical, All is Consciousness.

Ancient teachings of traditional Chinese Medicine say we are part of a Trigram which squarely places human kind between the twin fields of influence of heaven and earth. Heaven, Man, Earth make up the first of the sixty four tri-grams, making up the lexicon or library of the I-Ching made famous by ancient Chinese historical figure of Lao Tse. This is similarly stated in many other ancient traditions and school as well such as Indian Ayurveda. In Ayurveda mankind is described as a vessel, a pathway or conduit of communication between the twin male and female primordial influences of Purusha and Prakruti i.e. heaven and earth. The manifestation of the harmonious terrestrial and celestial forces are being disrupted, fractured and or separated by the Ego.

One Vedic teacher of mine described the common origin of all disease, illness and suffering as simply being separated from the direct personal knowledge of god consciousness by ego. We say there is a god for each kind of man or machine and the closest ordinary man comes to direct personal experience of god consciousness is in experience of pure or true essence. If there is a more or greater experience of god realization than this, we will have to get to the pure and true manifestation of undefiled essence to be able to see it! Normally, we don't talk of deities much, as work is better served by focusing on what is directly experienced and verifiable at any given time.

The Native American traditions portray or show us as "upright, two-leggeds, walking between Father Sky and Mother Earth in the company of all living beings." These traditions in their own way seek to explain and make use of the observed fact that we exist in the greater fields and energies of the world around us, that there is polarity either masculine or feminine, as characteristic of the interplay between these great forces. It is polarity, which is mirrored within our own makeup and constitutions. It is polarity – plus or minus, male or female, heaven or earth – that sets, establishes and differentiates the order, place and hierarchy and eventual function of all things. To the sub-atomic level everything has either polarity, or is made up of elements which do. It is this polarity which is the basis for electricity! Everything that there is, from solid matter to light, follows this principle.

Everything is electrical! The difference between things is found on the electromagnetic continuum, i.e., some particles or wave forms move relatively faster or slower in reference to one another and as these faster or slower particles or wave forms travel, they travel coherently and in predictable patterns or interference patterns called waves.

In the new Quantum physics, the traditional model of matter being made up of individual sub-atomic particles called atoms , neutrons, protons, quarks, all circling one another with 99 percent of their "orbits" being made up of empty space has gone by the wayside. There are new theories postulating that there are no "orbits" and there is NO "empty space!"

The organization of sub-atomic structure now appears to be seen more as "Wave" patterns with resonance, interference and affinity characteristics determining fundamental structure and organization. Our understanding is concurrent with this "new" view.

These waves have form and substance and affect or impact one another and create effects called harmonics and resonances and interference patterns which add to, take away from or vary the shape and action of the waves. Everything that exists is a by-product of these interactions, including us!

Our essence, being organic, our physicality, as well as everything that exists in our world, is energetic and electrical in this fashion. This is what Ayurveda refers to when it states, "Originating out of the formless, the primordial sound, vibration OM, originates all that there is." Om is or represents the primordial or original electrical vibrational nature of the universe and is a representation of everything. Everything that follows the primordial OM is but differentiations in this fundamental electrical nature of the universe.

Fields within fields, waves interacting with waves based on affinity principles and patterns generated by polarity and frequency, amplitude and all principles of the quantum atomic, electromagnetic world.

When we say "All is God, All is Energy, All is Electrical, All is Consciousness," we may be approximating the truth of our nature.

Premise #24: Energy precedes physiology.

There is no physicality or organic physiology, biology or chemistry without energy. Literally, energy in some form is the precursor to everything that is, ever was, will or might be.

Actually "Energy precedes Physiology" is only a part of a larger concept. This concept is derived from Ayurveda and relates to the original or "Cosmic" consciousness. As quoted from the book Lines, Wheels, Points and Specific Remedies by the same author, "Cosmic Consciousness preceding manifestation leads us to a formula.

Past actions or original inclinations, (In Thai called Kamma or Karma) precede energy elements, and energy elements precede physiology or matter elements. We could also say that acknowledgement precedes intention. Intention precedes extension and or affirmation. Affirmation precedes Action and action leads to manifestation."

Premise #25: The Cause of All Negative Emotion is Disruption of the Body's Energy System.

Negative emotions are symptoms of imbalance and or disruption in the Matrix Body or the body's energy system. These imbalances which can cause negative emotional symptoms can range from lack of harmony between the organs to excesses or deficiencies between the Chakra, or between the many, secondary and tertiary energy points, Lom, Marma, Lines, Nadi, Meridians., and others.

Imbalance is usually the result of some harmful influence originating either from outside the person or from within. Imbalance can also be the result of trauma and or discord and frustration in the expression of one's nature, especially in regard to sexual being.

Negative emotions can be both a cause and an effect of physical distortion and armoring of the tissue. Negative emotion can be released or corrected by balancing the body's energy system.

Premise #26: We can change physiology by affecting energy.

We can affect or cause changes in the body's, neurology, physiology and chemistry, even tissue states, by affecting energy. We can support or cause effects of either a negative or positive manner in the body by affecting the energy of the body. We can affect energy by changing physiology.

Premise #27: The body is a stress adaptive organism and vehicle for transformation.

Our machine's purpose is to be a vehicle for the spirit it has been said. However, the implication is a bit unclear. The body or machine carries us, our spirit or essence around like a glorified taxi? No! The body's job is first to host, then to affect the essence, literally to transform the essence to such a degree that not the essence eventually becomes the mind and controls the body. Further, the body develops the essence to a point of self-awareness and substance that will continue intact past the death of the body or life of the machine. One of the machine's abilities is to teach us that we are not machines! We are something else.

Premise #28 We are not the "Machine," nor are we the "Events" which happen to it!

We are not the sum of the events that occur to the machine (HBTM). We are not that which happens to us or around us. Although external events may influence our machines life and circumstances, essence occurs outside of the direct influence of transient events and is not identified as them.

When examining the patterns of disturbance and manifestations of negativity and the expression of negative emotions we commonly find that there is a "Story" which is cited as the cause or genesis of the negative occurrences or negative emotions whatever they might be. There is association with the story. The story may be held so strongly that virtually every significant part of life may be affected by and held against the template of this story.

A story is an EVENT. What happens to us is often of no more consciousness than rain storms or other natural phenomenon. But we take the emotions, especially the negative emotions which occur at the same time as the event to be real, to be definitive in some context and they are stored and nurtured becoming emotional templates that attract and gather all such similar "Stories" and events. Stories are interpreted according to the degree of similarity to the key trigger events and stories that set up the original energy imbalance. Often there was electrical imbalance before the events and or occurrence of the story which forever after is seen as the cause of the negative emotions!

For example, one client of mine with a twenty year history of neck and shoulder pain, when questioned about the history of her debilitating condition, told the story of an accident in a car which took place in a super market parking lot. She was backing up to pull out of her space and backed into another car, parked behind her. She was going no more than 5 miles and hour. However, she was surprised and felt her head move, followed by sharp pain. She was eventually medically diagnosed as having trauma to her neck called "Whiplash."

Going for various treatments over a period of twenty years not only appeared to not be helpful, but her condition also deteriorated to the point of disability. This was her status when she first came to my office. So in her interview, she relates this pivotal moment, event and her subsequent story. Mostly, she was trying to convince herself and, I am sure anyone around her, that her pain and disability were entirely justified having a clear origin.

However, as I looked at her from the point of view of someone who understands that energy precedes physiology and that pain and suffering are manifestations of negative emotions which are caused by disruptions in the body's energy field, I simply went on and started balancing points which should have had no impact on the story. After a couple of sessions, as we were sitting and discussing her level of pain after a treatment, she suddenly started relating a different story.

The new revised story did not begin in the parking lot! It began earlier in the day when she had a fuss or fight with a step-father who had accused her of being "irresponsible and lazy." This had caused her to become extremely upset and as she was pulling out of that parking spot, she was crying severely until the moment of impact! Now, literally as she sat there, I immediately treated her again for issues based on that fight. Using the words "irresponsible," and "lazy," and in less than five minutes she was pain free. Pain free for the first time in 20 years! No organic or structural corrections or alignments were done.

The format for the treatments I was giving her is what we call a general energy balancing. If, as her story would seem to say, the nature of her disability was the structural problems associated with this traumatic event and the subsequent tissue distortions and side effects, there really is no way that uncovering a root event relating to the event's negative emotions would help. Ending her disability would take more than simply balancing her energy. So, we concluded the cause of her pain and eventual disability was not the event, but rather, it was the negative emotions in place before the event which the event naturally fed into. The event was stored and catalogued and confirmed the negative emotions.

Once we resolved the electrical imbalance associated with the story, the story was no longer able to continue to cause the pain! It has been several years now since Ms. Betty's sessions and there has been no further recurrence of her original neck pain and she is no longer disabled. I guess from a "medical" point of view, it could be said that she just happened to have a spontaneous correction or remission for no apparent reason during our sessions! You be the judge.

Premise #29: Balance The Fields

One of our goals is to weaken the machine's electrical field dominance in relation to the field strength and influence of the essence. To be asleep means that the machine's field is dominant. The statement "to be awake" means that the essence field is dominant.

Premise #30: "I's" equal sources of inference.

One reason the machine's electrical field is so dominant is because of the accumulated interference wave patterns aggregated and stored in the tissues, organs and physical structures of the machine. The sum of these complex and mostly negative fields is like having one hundred random talk radio stations all broadcasting on the same frequency, at the same time and frequency – the frequency being that of the needful "Emergency Broadcast Frequency" of the essence or true nature. The proper agency or steward for that key frequency will have to come in and close down the pirate broadcast, or at least remove them to a less vital frequency/bandwidth. This action intentionally preserves the vital frequencies for more appropriate use.

Our emergency and urgent broadcast in this example is the direct, uncompromising communications from the essential self. We can't "get it," because we can't "hear it"!

These many stations broadcasting interference negatively affecting both the machine and possible work of the machine are the many "I's." "I's" equal sources of interference.

Premise #31: Everything about you is mechanical, except what is not!

The body entirely, the mind and spirit as well, is entirely mechanical, following cause and effect, affinity and repulsion and utilization of resources as any other mechanical or unconscious mechanism. For example, in classical Indian Medicine or Ayurveda, the mind is described as an organ and no more special than any other organ. There might be such a thing as essential nature or essence apart from the life of the machine, but only hypothetically and only possibly in a transformed machine of a self realized, trained, awakened and lucky individual.

Premise #32: All chronic disorder and disease in the machine is supported by negative emotion.

Considering "Premise #25: The Cause of All Negative Emotion is Disruption of the Body's Energy System. We then say the ultimate cause of all chronic disorder and disease is also a disruption of the body's energy system. Furthermore, disruptions of the body's energy system, past or current, support disorder and disease. So these types of disruptions are both cause and support for imbalance at the same time. We can only surmise that correcting this energy issue will have an immediate and profound effect on both the current condition and the future development, course or severity of it.

Premise #33: Where it hurts it ain't!

Our ability to understand and correctly determine the nature of pain and/or source of pain within us is severely limited. It is entirely subject to distortion at almost every level of perception. Neurologists, inform us as to the phenomena of the pathological reflex arc for example in physical pain issues. For example, in the case of a common headache, the pain is obviously in some part of the head, giving any reasonable person the thought or feeling that there is something wrong in their head – Not true!

In most cases the pain is actually a referral pain from some localized disturbance or trigger point (area of low oxygen and high neurologic activity) which could be located possibly in any or several different locations all the way down to the upper torso! Distortion and misinterpretation of the nature, source and cause of any pain is the norm, not the exception. Also, pain can be originating from any part or multiple parts of us at any time and these connections are generally not easily observed. The pain can be physical but nonspecific in the sense that it is a referral pain from some other area of the body under stress. The pain can be emotional, it can be symptomatic of an energy disturbance. It can be in a sense, a memory from an unresolved traumatic issue arising from the past or layers of all the above.

In simple terms, the best thing pain represents is a symptom and indicator that something needs attention. However, in the absence of some overt trauma like a wound, pain, in and of itself, has little specific meaning. It's like an idiot light on the car's dashboard. It means, have a look under the hood and always do a general diagnostic. Always check everything fundamental before deciding what the pain might mean. Whatever it means, it means something only in the context of the complete functioning of the person and that person's life.

Premise #34: Psychological, Mental illness and Negative emotions are the same and have the same causes.

So-called psychological illnesses and mental diseases of the mind do not exist apart from us as symptoms of disruptions of the body's energy system. The modern Western psychology or the fields of psychiatry and psychology have missed the boat. Modern psychiatry seeks to define mental illness as the result of purely chemical imbalances in the brain and completely ignores the causative factors of disruptions of the body's energy system. Using this model has been an almost complete failure to the many persons referred for various treatments. The chemical imbalance model does nothing good for patients and is a blatant push to develop drug and chemical dependencies for producing income and control over persons without their consent. There is no known test which can medically or scientifically correlate any specific mental illness or condition with a specific chemical deficiency. Most, if not all mental illnesses, are described as aggregates of symptoms of negative emotions. We treat the negative emotions to support mental health.

A story about healing...

I have thought on this bothersome incident for over 25 years now and finally have the answer that was given to me right back then! To understand my question and issue I think it will be beneficial to share the story as I witnessed it.

The year was 1982. It was a hot Saturday afternoon in April in Nongkam, Thailand, and I was in a group class practicing what the Thai call "Wai Khruu." The Wai Khruu we were practicing that day was about paying respect to three teachers and four directions and is a physical form similar to Tai Chi or Chi Gung.

If you have ever been to southern Thailand in April you know it was HOT! The weather averaged about 100 degrees daily with about 100 percent humidity! Miserably hot, but, hey life goes on, and we were in school and had to practice regardless. The class was out doors under a shaded pavilion type of area. As we were practicing, I noticed a boy of about 13 to 14 years of age slowly walking into the compound with a severe limp. Even at a distance I could see he was in some great pain. He walked over close to where we were practicing and sat down on a bench there.

I excused myself and walked over to him to see what was the matter. As I got close to him, I could see that his leg was broken – a nasty compound fracture with the bone visibly protruding from the skin! More than this, it was immediately apparent that his leg was severely infected. It was swollen badly enough that the skin was splitting and, well, just looked awful as I'm sure you can imagine. I immediately went to the head Master Phaa Khruu to interrupt him and to basically tell him what was going on. I was sure at that moment that the boy needed emergency medical treatment and also knew the nearest Western clinic was over two hours away by bus!

Phaa Kruu asked me what was the matter. I explained about the boy who he could clearly see, who was now lying on the bench. He told me to go back to class! I said, "But Phaa Khruu, this boy needs medical help, emergency medical help." He again told me to mind my own business and go back to my place in class. This time I was adamant, as I was sure he did not understand the severity of the boy's situation at all! So I pleaded and said that I would take him to the hospital at my own expense, but he needed antibiotics or he could die. Now at this point I should inform you, as you probably don't know, that the school I was in was a traditional oriental Medical school famous for producing Doctors of Traditional Thai Medicine! Phaa Khruu Samaii was not just the Head Master he was the 36th generation of Grand Masters leading that school! So, here I am, the only western student, freaking out during an emergency and basically demanding Western antibiotics, as in "Real" medicine. Phaa Khruu told me not to worry that as soon as the class finished he would go to see to the boy but if I wanted to remain a student I had to stop interrupting and get back to class.

I have to say in that moment there was a critical decision that has affected my life ever since. I surrendered and did as he instructed. Phaa Khruu said the issue was between him and god and that if it was god's will that help manifest for the boy, then it would. However, being hysterical was not the way to manifest healing for the boy.

After class, about 20 minutes later, he walked over to the boy with me about one inch behind him. He came close and looked at the boy and his leg. He then lightly shook him into awareness and when his eyes focused, Phaa Khruu asked the boy "What is the Matter?"

I was amazed, I mean, he had a bone sticking out of a huge and oozing leg. What kind of question was this and why was he asking in the first place? I mean, it was clear someone needed to take charge and just scoop this boy up and run like the wind to a real hospital, and even so, he might not make it. But, here we are asking silly questions.

The boy looked up and said he had broken his leg in a motorcycle accident and knowing of the school (Buddhai Sawan) had walked from his wreck seeking help. Phaa Kruu then asked him "What can we do for you?" Again, I thought to myself, "Insane! What is going on here?" It was surreal. Up to this moment I would have sworn that the school and community I was living and studying in was one of the most compassionate and gentle, loving environments I had ever been in and all of a sudden, without warning, the first very serious case I see and they are being mean. What did it mean?

The conversation continued.

"Please help me," the boy answered.
"Help you what?" Phaa Khruu replied.
"Fix my leg." the boy answered.
"Have you paid respect today?" Phaa Khruu then asked.

Meaning, have you paid respect or homage to the Buddha today? Most Thai are Buddhist and the term Buddha is synonymous with god or spirit.

"No," the boy answered, hanging his head, and then, somewhat sadly it seemed. "No."

"We will help you after you pay respect," Phaa Khruu answered. "When you're done paying respect, come see me and I will help you in the name of the Buddha."

I turned to phaa Khruu, incredulous at the further delay and apparent lack of concern to my eyes and said, "Phaa Khruu, even if this boy could pay respect, his leg is broken. He can no longer walk. How will he do this?"

He looked at me and said "Well, then. Carry him if that is what it takes." He then proceeded to walk away without another word.

Oh my god. I stood there transfixed not really knowing proper cause of action, "What do I do, now?" I asked myself.

I was in anguish looking at this poor child, but something inside asked me to do as I was told. After a moment, I went over to the Altar and picked up some Joss or incense and brought it back. I gently picked up the boy and helped carry him over to the first of three altars. At Buddhai Sawan, there were three principle altars and the ritual was to go to each, ask for a blessing and burn a stick or two of incense as a way of paying respect.

We made our way a bit quickly, as I was still thinking it possible for me to make off to the highway with the boy and hitch a ride to town. Anyway, we came back to the pavilion and Phaa Khruu walks back and once again asks the boy what he wants. The boy says the same thing again, and asks him to help him. Phaa Khruu says that he can not help, but all help comes from the spirit and he would assist the boy. He then placed his hand on the boys head and told him to be still, as he was writhing and clearly uncomfortable. The boy immediately calmed and stopped moving. Phha Khruu told him to close his eyes, which he did. Phaa Khruu said to relax and the boy seemed to do this for the first time since walking in. However, he was still sweating profusely and was very, red in the face.

Phaa Khruu went over to the altar and obtained some "Blessing Oil" from it in a small bottle. It was thick and yellowish, smelling of Jasmine. He then went to the boy and touched him several times in different points on his body while reciting a prayer or Mantra. I could not tell what he was saying but it was short and repetitive. He then took the bottle back to the Altar and appeared finished. As he was working for about 5 minutes, the boys complexion evened out and he apparently settled into a deep sleep. "Or Coma," I thought to myself! Phaa Khruu asked for me and another to ease the boy onto a mat by the wall and let him sleep. Again I asked about taking him to a hospital, again I was refused. I was told it was his Karma, and if he died it was not to be my concern. He had come to the school for Phaa Khruu to fix him and Phaa Khruu was the responsible one. I placed a bandage over the exposed bone to keep the flies out of the wound.

I sat by the boy the balance of the day and night, he seldom moved or showed much of life. Once in a while, I would check his pulse and it was there and steady. He slept like this for 2 full days.

On the early morning of the third day, I was asleep nearby when the boy stirred and woke up asking for water. I jumped up and got him a glass of water. He looked completely different. He was weakened, but not dire. I looked at his leg and the swelling was reduced and there was a scab. There was no sign of the bone at all! From this point, the boy continued to get better. He ate and was chatty with the other students and children there.

Fourteen days after he first dragged himself into the compound, he was up on his feet trying to play a game of Tak Kraw with the kids. If you knew Tak Kraw you would know its like ultimate Hackey Sack, a game like volleyball played with your feet! I was watching and more than a little in wonder when Phaa Khruu comes out and angrily calls the boy over. The boy sheepishly walks over and Phaa Khruu asks him "How's the leg?" The boy looks down and wiggles his toes before saying, "I guess it's ok." Pha Khruu then points out toward the gate and says "Then off you go! Don't forget to pay respect every day."

The boy turned, shook my hand, and said "Khap Khun Khrap (Thank You)," turned and walked out. I never saw him again.

Life went on and classes took up much space. Learning acupuncture, Thai Yoga, Martial arts at the same time in a traditional school takes everything you can dig up to stay on top, especially when you have some difficulties with the language.

About a month later, I was speaking with Phaa Khruu, who spoke excellent English, having obtained a degree from Oxford University in England. I asked him what was the essence of healing, what was the minimum required to create a healing occurrence. I still had the recent events in my mind. He explained it like this: "Anthony, a person comes to you for help and asks you for help. You agree to help them. They get well. That's it.

Everything else is just window dressing."

Can you see why this event has weighed on my mind? Through my continued education and clinical practice I have maintained this question: How to do this? I have over the years come to understand, that I have always, that we have always, had the keys to healing and they are sooo simple, so elegant and easy.

For other SomaVeda® Integrated Traditional Therapies
books, DVD, Home Study Courses and more, visit:
WWW.BeardedMedia.Com

For ongoing live courses and training's in Thai Yoga and
Holistic Health Provider education visit:
www.ThaiYogaCenter.Com

9 781886 338241   52088

www.ingramcontent.com/pod-product-compliance
Lightning Source LLC
Chambersburg PA
CBHW031523270326
41930CB00006B/501